HOW TO BE A
TERRIBLE
NURSE

HOW TO BE A TERRIBLE NURSE

10 DOCTOR'S ORDERS TO ACHIEVE PEAK LOUSINESS

KOLYA K. JAXSON, MD

TITL VENTURES

How To Be A Terrible Nurse is a work of fiction.

Names, characters, places and incidents are the products of the author's imagination or are used fictitiously. Any resemblance to actual events, locales, or persons, living or dead, is entirely coincidental.

Copyright © 2018 by Kolya K. Jaxson
All rights reserved.

Printed in the United States of America

ISBN-13: 978-1986003810
ISBN-10: 1986003817

TABLE OF CONTENTS

ORDER #1: *Stop Caring* 3

ORDER #2: *Stop Thinking* 5

ORDER #3: *Neglect Yourself* 7

ORDER #4: *Complain* 11

ORDER #5: *Resent Doctors* 13

ORDER #6: *Never Be Gentle* 15

ORDER #7: *Be Unreliable* 17

ORDER #8: *Be Haphazard With Medications* 19

ORDER #9: *Practice Cannibalism* 23

ORDER #10: *Burn Out* 25

Epilogue 27

About the Author 29

About TITL Ventures 31

*"Let us never consider ourselves finished nurses....
we must be learning all of our lives."*

— Florence Nightingale

Hey.

Why are you reading this? Don't you have something, ANYTHING, better or more important to do?

Let me answer for you. No, you don't.

Allow me to introduce myself. I'm a doctor. I wrote a wildly successful book called "How To Be A Terrible Doctor." It's crushed every publishing record, caused climate change, broke the Internet, and was even nominated for a Nobel Peace Prize. But I don't pay attention to such things.

My life's work is as a teacher and spiritual guide. That's where you come in.

Presumably, you are a nurse. And you need help. You're trying your hardest but coming up short, failing to live up to your potential.

You've consulted with fellow nurses. Followed their Instagram. Watched their YouTube channels and listened to their podcasts. Even talked to some in person. And yet it's still not enough.

So why listen to a doctor instead?

Over the last twenty years I've worked with many many nurses. Most have been average; a select few have been truly awful. The best of the worst know that healthcare is a sacred union between doctor and nurse, and that combining -1 + -1= -3, results otherwise unattainable for either party alone.

The Doctor's Orders that follow will lead you to this Promised Land. Listen and learn, let's begin.

ORDER #1
STOP CARING

The absolute foundation of nursing of any variety whatsoever is compassion.

Nurses bear witness to the full spectrum of human experience across all domains. Age. Social status. Race. Religion. Agony. Ecstasy. Victory and defeat.

Far from being a passive spectator, nurses are crucial to the arc of the patient's journey. In assessing the physical, emotional, and spiritual status of their patients, nurses deduce the essence of that individual and accordingly apply their own unique talents to guide patients with tender care toward wellness and peace.

It is a process of integration, sharing, and deeply personal connection between souls invested in common goals.

Now, to have any hope of becoming a Terrible Nurse, you MUST divest yourself of any and all traces of caring and compassion. If you are unable or unwilling to do so, please stop reading now and return to your present life. Because any further efforts will be futile and the remaining Orders will be impotent.

Still with me? Then we shall proceed.

Fortunately, there are as many ways to kill compassion and caring as there are stars in the sky. One size does not fit all, so you will need to determine the best approaches particular to your situation. Start low and go slow. Consider yourself chronically NPO in this matter. Bingeing on a smorgasbord will only end badly. Here are some starting sips:

INDIFFERENCE is a fine place to begin. By simply not giving a rat's ass one way or another about much of anything going on with your patient you've conserved energy and partially disengaged from the therapeutic relationship.

Wrong food tray arrived? Yawn. Procedure rescheduled? Meh. Gown and linens soiled? Whatever.

A strong baseline practice of indifference will pave the way to other effective approaches.

LETHARGY feeds off of laziness tendencies to chip away at compassion. Answering a call bell, contacting a patient's family member or doing a teach back involve effort! Doesn't anyone understand how much work these things entail? Now please excuse me while I take the elevator down ten floors and walk 150 feet outside to have a cigarette at the smoker's oasis.

ANIMOSITY transforms resentment toward patients into active destruction of empathy. You mean I have to delay my lunch break because that jerk decided to have a cardiac arrest? Look how pretty/handsome their spouse is. Why am I stuck with such a loser? Maybe my back wouldn't hurt so much if you just lost 200 pounds. Right now!

The list of options goes on and on. Seek and you will find the ones that meet your needs.

ORDER #2
STOP THINKING

Becoming a nurse requires a difficult curriculum of diverse coursework. There are core studies in biology, anatomy and physiology, pathology and pharmacology. Procedural education such as insertion of intravenous and urinary catheters, sterile dressing changes, proper administration of medications and physical examination skills round out a rigorous syllabus.

Furthermore, it is necessary to rotate among many different clinical disciplines such as medical, surgical, pediatric, obstetric, oncologic and behavioral units. Such a dizzying array of facts, figures and technical capabilities mandates that the conscientious nurse study hard to obtain knowledge, develop keen observation skills in the clinical arena and marry those powers to thoughtfully apply them to the specific patients before them.

The Terrible Nurse can't be bothered with all that.

Sure, you did what you had to in order to get through nursing school and get your license. But once you do that, at least if you truly want to be a Terrible Nurse (and you do, don't you?) it's Operation Shutdown for your brain.

How you stop thinking can take different forms.

At a minimum, letting your current knowledge get old and fester will do. Avoid reading, classes, or updates in your field. Yes, CEUs will be necessary to stay on the job, but choose these based on ease of completion, not relevance or quality. If they can be obtained at a sunny destination while you lounge on the beach, all the better.

By not learning anything new, forgetting what you already know, and using outdated practices, you'll get worse and worse.

Blind obedience works like a charm as well.

Doctors and pharmacists, they went through even more schooling than you did. And they get paid more. So why should you think on their behalf?

Don't question an insulin dose when the patient is NPO, a possible drug allergy, or abnormal labs that nobody seems to know or care about. Tune out and turn off, know your place and leave the mental gymnastics for others.

On the flip side, hell-bent defiance with a lone wolf mentality can also serve the Terrible Nurse well.

In these instances rather than engaging with the patient, doctor, therapist, pharmacist or anyone else trying to help you adapt to a delicate or complex circumstance, you will stick to your guns and carry out your mission as you see fit.

Blood pressure or heart rate slightly low for your liking? Hold meds despite reassurances from the cardiologist. Too many bedpan visits for the patient on diuretics? Demand a Foley, or better yet, put one in and worry about getting an order later. A shadowy phantom verbal order from an unsuspecting nocturnist or surgical PA works nicely. Grandma's sundowning tiring you out? Snow her with benzos after browbeating the hospitalist into submission.

Stop thinking and start living!

ORDER #3
NEGLECT YOURSELF

Nursing is a service profession that involves helping and doing work on behalf of and for others. Patients and their family members, doctors, and administrators demand much from bedside nurses. Long hours, the emotional roller coaster of life and death situations, physically and mentally exhausting work and frequent ingratitude can make a tough job to begin with seemingly impossible.

The best nurses understand that you cannot give what you do not yourself have. By cultivating personal health and wellness in themselves they are able to demonstrate compassion, understanding, hope in hardship, and be a trusted role model.

The Terrible Nurse cackles at such fairy tales.

Where to begin?

A general framework for comprehensive wellness consists of physical, emotional, mental, and spiritual health. Neglecting a few of these components will drop you down a few pegs, but if you REALLY want to suck as a nurse pay attention and check off as many of the following boxes as you can.

Physical:

1. **Eating**—Eat too much or too little. Eat the wrong things at the wrong times and in the wrong places. You'll feel fatigued and irritable or bloated and sleepy, either of which will translate into poor care. Walking into a vomiting patient's room with a mouthful of General Tso's chicken is one such example.
2. **Sleeping**—Less is more in terms of dulling your intellect, frazzling your nerves and making you generally miserable. Double or triple down on your caffeine too while you're at it, OK?
3. **Exercise.** HA! No further comment necessary.

Emotional:

Maintain toxic relationships. Spouse or S.O. running around on you? Blame yourself and feel worthless and guilty. Adult kids play video games and smoke weed all day, won't move out or get a job? Subsidize them without questions, indefinitely.

Mental:

This has already been covered extensively in ORDER #2, STOP THINKING. However, to really crater your IQ, alcohol and drug use act as a force multiplier and will also ruin other areas of your life, so strongly consider adding on this modality.

Spiritual:

See no larger purpose in your professional duties, focusing on the flaws in each tree and never appreciating the beauty and significance of the larger forest. Disimpacting an elderly hospice patient struggling for comfort in their final days? Puh-leeze.

Neglect yourself well and you will naturally begin to neglect others. Truth.

ORDER #4
COMPLAIN

Through our journey thus far we have very clearly established how hard it is to be a nurse. Much of the work is tedious, dirty, and thankless. The star nurse understands that these tasks, routine and unfulfilling as they may be in the moment, lay the foundation for later positive outcomes that would be impossible otherwise.

As an example, hourly rounding brings visibility and reassurance and allows evaluation of such things as pain, position, potty and possessions. Anticipating needs and providing early interventions such as analgesics, turning patients to prevent bedsores, toileting, and refilling a water cup are simple yet powerful actions that bring immediate comfort, demonstrate concern, and prevent patient decline.

The Terrible Nurse fights tooth and nail against such an administrative straightjacket.

As an outstanding mathematician, (s)he will churn out data with computer like speed and sophistication, overwhelming their poor supervisors.

"Hourly rounding? I have four patients. FOUR PATIENTS! And I'm working a TWELVE-HOUR shift. So FOUR PATIENTS times TWELVE HOURS is, like, FORTY-EIGHT HOURS of work! And when I go into that room, trust me, it's not like there's only one thing to do. You yourself are telling me to assess the FOUR P's."

"So FOUR P's times FOUR PATIENTS times TWELVE HOURS is ONE HUNDRED AND NINETY TWO things to do!"

Having laid out the basic statistics and setting the proper tone, launch into a litany of piggybacked complaints. It's unnecessary for them to be related to the current topic, and truthfully, feel free to pull in things completely irrelevant to your specific job, workplace, or even nursing in general. Build momentum and roll on.

Criticize the EMR and how long documentation takes, how there aren't enough computers on the ward, and how slow the ones you do have are. For good measure, throw in a sly reference regarding social media blocking filters.

Complain about how arrogant and condescending the surgeons are, and how nit picky they are about their silly little spine procedures.

Dis the CNA's and PCT's as lazy, stupid, and disrespectful, and comment on how instead of making your life easier, they actually make it much harder since you have to triple check everything they do and usually end up redoing it anyway. Before your stunned supervisor can respond, go for the left hook knockout punch by immediately insisting that they hire many more techs, despite no obvious budget to do so.

Civil discussions over valid concerns such as workplace violence and safety, compensation, mandatory overtime, and appropriate staffing ratios are not for you, the Terrible Nurse, to consider. Stick to voicing bitter personal gripes without offering solutions. It's what you do best.

ORDER #5
RESENT DOCTORS

Let's revisit ORDER #4, COMPLAIN, for a moment. Before the spawn of an actual complaint, there must first exist a source; a spark of indignation, grievance, grudge, dislike, objection, displeasure, insult, slight, or other ill will that provides the seeds of discontent that bloom into a stinking bouquet of complaints. Without question, a most fruitful source of these seeds (and their fertilizer) will be doctors.

Doctors dictate and direct many of the duties nurses find themselves tasked with. Whether it is the frequency of vital signs, wound care regimens, enema administration, neurologic checks, ambulating patients, flushing cerumen from elderly ears, hunting down hospital records, completing operative or procedural consents, or teaching fingersticks and insulin to a new diabetic, most of what a nurse's shift looks like is a direct result of some or many doctor's whims.

To transform into a Terrible Nurse and carry out these commands with spite and malicious intent will be much enhanced by hating on doctors. Here's how.

Compare and contrast. Doctors are either smarter or dumber than you. Fatter or fitter. Nicer or meaner. They dress sharply or look like slobs. They may be quite socially adept or inept. Whatever the case may be, doctors tell you what to do and how to do it, and get paid boatloads of cash to do so.

Focus on the personal differences between yourself and individual doctors and turn these into feelings of superiority or inferiority. Let these feelings stew. After a time, you will begin to despise doctors for their talents or shortcomings and equate their professional judgments and performance with factors that are purely cosmetic or unrelated to patient care. This mindset will contaminate your perspective and performance and transfer to your patients, as your scorn for their doctors undermines confidence and hope regarding treatment plans. And isn't that the point?

ORDER #6
NEVER BE GENTLE

Illness and malaise often heighten sensitivity to the constant barrage of stimuli life throws at us. The considerate nurse intuitively understands this and will seek to limit or tone down harsh exposures to their patients.

Intolerance to heat or cold? A fan or warm blanket to the rescue! Room too bright? Let me draw the curtains or dim the lights. Discomfort in bed? I'll reposition you and bring some extra pillows.

These are but a few examples of how to lessen harmful impacts and make patients feel better. Understanding a patient's reduced abilities allows the good nurse to gently soften discomfort in any form and speed the recovery of their patients.

What wimps.

Um, did someone forget that nursing is a full contact profession?

Hear me out.

If you're planning to survive in this game, you need to be tough. Tough and rough. Loud and proud. Large and in charge.

Just whose doormat do you think you are? Start giving an inch to cater to others and they'll take a marathon from your soul.

If you don't assert yourself with force, get used to your wants and needs being trampled. Here's how to avoid that.

Amplify everything.

Your voice should be loud at all times. Assume everybody is hearing impaired and shout. Unsolicited, strongly advertise your political beliefs. These practices will project authority and confidence.

Your movements and your movement of others should be fast, furious, and frantic. Rush around in chaos for no apparent reason, tug and pull patients around indelicately and use wild hand gestures to convey frustration and impatience.

Big up your appearance. Wear neon scrubs, logoed bandanas or surgical caps. Slather on gallons of perfume or cologne and sport every karat of bling you can buy borrow or steal.

If you have ink, figure out how to display it prominently. Full sleeve arm tats of demons, skulls, and warlocks or a neck that looks like a Chinese novel are just what elderly patients love and most respect best, so don't disappoint them.

Always max out your surrounding environment as well. Shake rattle and roll equipment. Play inappropriate music at an intolerable volume. Crank the thermostat to create an icebox or a sweat lodge. Maintain utter darkness or blinding light.

Terrible Nurses announce and impose their will. And so will you.

ORDER #7
BE UNRELIABLE

Competence and consistency go hand in hand. In order to be considered a capable nurse, or really a capable anything, requires demonstration of a stable pattern of behaviors and outputs that define performance.

The buzzword "hardwired" comes to mind. Managers will often use this term to describe practices that have been repeated so often that they become virtually automatic, part of the DNA and culture of the individual nurse and their parent organization.

Hourly rounding. Barcode scanning of medications. Two factor identity authentication. And so on and so forth.

To be a Terrible Nurse, you must not only be inconsistent, you must be inconsistently inconsistent.

It's important to keep people guessing and unsure regarding your personality, temperament, stability, skills, motivation, knowledge, commitment, work ethic and any other element of your being.

In short, make dependability and predictability in all matters joker wild cards in the deck of your life.

Arrive late or early for work when you are scheduled, and for good measure occasionally no-show. Once in a while, when you are knowingly not scheduled to work, show up under the premise that you are and make a scene about how someone (once again) screwed up the schedule.

When charting, mix it up. Document by exception when your shifts are eventful, leaving no trace of any meaningful events regarding your patients. Conversely, generate a full-length novel of notes on your stable patients awaiting nursing home placement. Document the caliber, frequency, and odor of their stools. Record every individual morsel of food consumed from the meal tray, including an itemized calorie count even if, perhaps especially if, the patient's appetite is voracious.

When calling doctors, strive for a bipolar approach. Call them relentlessly and with a sense of urgency for stool softeners, p.r.n. acetaminophen, and to report results of routine labs, all the better when they are stone cold normal. On the flip side, be nonchalant about reaching out when the shit hits, or is about to hit, the fan. Steadily dropping blood pressure, increasing agitation or lethargy, or a potentially dangerous medication are good examples of things to minimize or blow off completely.

Change up your style of communication as well. Adopt a militant adherence to template tools such as SBAR when brief normal conversation will do. Alternate with completely unstructured vague casual conversations punctuated by impossible requests. For example: "Hi? It's Erin on 4 Tower? My patient (note—don't give name, age, condition, context) is a little short of breath? Could we maybe, like, try some Versed?"

Navigate your course to becoming a Terrible Nurse by being all over the map.

ORDER #8
BE HAPHAZARD WITH MEDICATIONS

Most nurses spend a great deal of time dealing with medications. Whether it occurs at an ED, hospital ward, clinic, PACU, urgent care center, nursing home or rehab facility, this endeavor is usually a core function of nursing.

For starters, pretty much every patient is on a medication or twenty. Probably closer to fifty when you add in all the OTC vitamins, supplements, antacids, cough/cold/sinus combinations and other ineffective crap that people take.

You may well be called upon to do what is affectionately known as "medication reconciliation." What a pleasant sounding phrase. It even rhymes. It conjures up happy images of all these prescriptions overcoming their differences and incompatibilities and living together in a perfect drug utopia melting pot. Blue and red pills cohabitating, tablets and capsules vacationing together, IV drips and transdermal patches working in harmony side by side.

This, of course, is a fantasy.

First off, most patients don't know what the hell they're taking (if they are, which they probably aren't, or at least not correctly,) why they're taking it, and how much or how often.

"Well, there's a pill for sugar. Then there's the tiny round yellow one that has the number 62 on it. There's some inhalers my lung doctor told me to use, but they cost $400 so I stopped them. And sometimes I'll take my wife's insulin if I ate too much ice cream."

Sigh.

Who are you kidding? Do you really think you can get to the bottom of this mess and clear things up? Not a chance.

The legendary Chinese General Sun-Tzu said: "To win without fighting, this is best."

Here's how, Terrible Nurse:

1. Copy and paste old lists. You can probably find these somewhere. Whether it's a week, a month or a year old, take them as unquestioned gospel. Do not verify or update the list with patients, pharmacies, family or doctor's offices.

2. Accept uncertainty. Look alike or sound alike meds? Just roll with your gut on it. What's so different about Maxalt and Maxipime? Florastor and Florinef? Doxepin and Klonopin?

3. Ignore therapeutic substitutions/duplications. Taking Prilosec and Protonix? Cool. Motrin and Advil? Awesome! Zocor and Pravachol? Epic.

Mucking up the med list is a good start but it's child's play compared to the damage you can do by actually administering meds.

Give meds too early or too late. For nauseated or uncooperative patients, completely quit efforts to get their pills down, or prioritize useless and trivial meds (simethicone, anyone?) over cardiovascular or Parkinson's agents. Hold meds that scare you by claiming that they were refused.

The Holy Grail of course is the beloved p.r.n. Supposedly Latin for *pro re nata*, or as necessary, it truly stands for PER RN. Meaning, per RN mood, patient load, hassle factor, disdain or affection for patient, convenience, and other factors.

The first step is to get access to p.r.n. orders. Make your doctors understand that it is in their interest to give you free reign to treat patients as you see fit. Demand p.r.n.'s for insomnia, for pain, for bowels, for anxiety, for nausea, for fever. Get nasal saline spray and artificial tears. Nystatin power for the folds, nooks, crannies and crevices. Barrier cream. Benadryl for itching, Meclizine for dizziness. Nitroglycerin. BP meds. And always: benzos and antipsychotics for agitation. Always.

Don't forget that oxygen is a drug too! Get the green light and slap it on, titrating to your heart's content between 0.5 and 3.3 L. So what if room air sats are normal?

After securing your stockpile of ammunition, fire away with reckless abandon. In general, strive to over or under medicate. Chastise post-op ortho patients who are "always on the call button" and "watching the clock," and suggest that they have an addiction problem when your offer of a 325mg acetaminophen suppository is met with a blank stare. Be quick to administer IV hydralazine for a BP of 157/93 after abruptly awakening a patient at 3:26am for 6 am vitals.

If you really want to be bold, double down by administering multiple p.r.n.'s followed with a "one time dose" requested chaser from the doctor. A good example would be the frightened and anxious demented patient who has already gotten benzos, narcotics, antihistamines and antipsychotics, but is still getting on your nerves. Just one more IM or IV (fill in the blank) please?

With enough practice you'll master the cookbook of bitches brews that will tame your patients and bring you peace.

ORDER #9
PRACTICE CANNABALISM

You know that saying about how nurses eat their young? Meaning that they don't support, mentor, teach, guide or otherwise nurture new nurses, and sometimes even actively act cruelly or vindictively toward them? Bad nurses do that. Terrible Nurses don't just dine on their babies. They chow down on the whole damn family.

Why selectively channel negative energy and attitude to just the young? Sure, they're a ripe target. Insecure and impressionable, lacking in confidence and real life experience, a few well-placed daggers on your part can scar them for life. By all means unleash your wicked wrath on these vulnerable sheep.

But don't stop there. Don't slack off and keep your poisonous personality and evil charms restricted to this tiny segment of the nursing species.

Lash out in every manner and direction. As alluded to previously, young nurses will get condescension, be attacked for their mistakes and naiveté, and be subjected to a general attitude of "They sure don't make them like they used to," or " When I was your age…" followed by whatever fictitious nonsense your selective memory conjures up.

Senior nurses will get criticized for being too slow, senile, outdated, infirmed, or otherwise "well past their prime."

Nurse administrators will get ragged on for being out of touch with bedside clinical practices, too stingy with budgets and too harsh with assignments.

If you're a surgical nurse, rip on your medical colleagues as sloppy, chaotic and undisciplined. Medical nurses, call out your surgical peeps as superficial airheads doing brainless and monotonous assembly line work.

Primary care nurses? Sniffle and sneeze princesses. Geriatric nurses? Wipe and dipe queens.

Any nurse that is not you deserves the full measure of your scorn, spite, gossip and sabotage.

Cannibalism: Breakfast (and lunch, and dinner) of Champions!

ORDER #10
BURN OUT

Congratulations! Here we are at ORDER #10, the last of our steps to becoming a Terrible Nurse. In many ways burnout takes care of itself, requiring little effort on your part. Many of the risks for burnout are deeply embedded in the nursing profession, almost to the point that a good dictionary definition for burnout could just say, "Being a nurse."

Mismatches in workload and control, lack of appropriate rewards, loss of a sense of positive connection with others, and a perceived lack of fairness lead to the hallmark symptoms of emotional exhaustion, depersonalization and treating others cynically, and reduced feelings of personal accomplishment. Following the first nine Orders in this manual will pour gas on the pilot light and virtually assure burnout. So that there is no margin for error though, follow these recommendations to nail the coffin shut.

1. Work too much. Do doubles, chase differentials for nights, weekends, and holidays. Always be first on the list for call-ins. Do

agency work despite lengthy travel, unpredictable environments, and unpleasant assignments. Fool yourself into thinking that you can sustain this pace indefinitely despite clear negative consequences to your health and relationships.

2. Avoid hobbies or other outside interests. Maintain a one-dimensional view of yourself and your place in the world. Working all the time helps to reinforce this, but is not essential. If you aren't a workaholic, on your off hours do mindless things like zoning out in front of a screen, eating out of boredom and depression or sleeping all the time (also out of boredom or depression.) Never take vacations, but if you must, park your sorry ass at a campground or beach, immobilize yourself for a week, preferably getting drunk daily, as you ask yourself what purpose you have in life.

3. Think, feel, and act as if you are entirely alone in your experience and there is no one who can understand and nothing that can help your situation. Maintain hopelessness at all costs and never consider let alone seek assistance.

Having thus burned out, the Terrible Nurse retires on the job: barely managing to show up, doing the absolute minimum, taking long breaks, disappearing for hours, offering little to no ideas, and being the first one out the door.

Make that person you.

EPILOGUE

Well, there you have it. The blueprint for your dreams, the feast to feed your appetite for destruction.

Heed these Orders and nothing can prevent you from becoming a Terrible Nurse.

How can I be so sure?

Because I'm a Terrible Doctor, and I said so.

ABOUT THE AUTHOR

Kolya K. Jaxson is a physician in New York.
He respects and admires nurses tremendously.

ABOUT TITL VENTURES

TITL Ventures is a global lifestyle syndicate.

www.ingramcontent.com/pod-product-compliance
Lightning Source LLC
Chambersburg PA
CBHW030101230526
45471CB00003B/1199